An Introduction to

TRANSCENDENTAL MEDITATION

Improve Your Brain Functioning,
Create Ideal Health,
and Gain Enlightenment
Naturally, Easily, and Effortlessly

Robert Keith Wallace, PhD and Lincoln Akin Norton

Dharma Publications

ISBN 978-0-9972207-0-4

Library of Congress Control Number: 2016901661

DharmaPublications.com

Dharma Publications, Fairfield, IA

Contents

FOR
MAHARISHI MAHESH YOGI

Preface

Keith and I were fortunate enough to have met Maharishi Mahesh Yogi relatively early in his travels around the world. Keith began meditating in 1964 and I started in 1966. We became teachers of the Transcendental Meditation® (TM®) technique in 1969 in Rishikesh, India, where we studied with Maharishi on the banks of the Ganges.

The purpose of this book is to serve as a basic introduction and to answer some of the most commonly asked questions about TM.

Transcendental Meditation is taught as a course, beginning with an introductory and preparatory lecture and a personal interview with the teacher. You then learn to meditate during personal one-on-one instruction with your teacher, followed by three group meetings, each only about an hour to an hour and a half long. After you have learned the practice from your teacher, the group meetings are extremely helpful because they give you a chance to hear a variety of experiences, many of which you will eventually have yourself.

There are over 165 locations in the United States where you can learn Transcendental Meditation, with about 500 active teachers. It should, therefore, not be too difficult to find a nearby center so that you can begin to have the experience of transcending. (See the website TM.org to find the teacher nearest you.)

It cannot be emphasized enough that Transcendental Meditation is not a religion, not a philosophy, not a belief system, and not a form of self-hypnosis. The practice of TM draws upon the natural ability of the human mind to transcend the deepest level of the thinking process and ultimately experience the source of thought, beyond mind, senses, intellect and ego. Regular transcending through the practice of the TM technique brings enormous benefits into daily activity. The experience may appear to be abstract until you practice this simple and effortless technique yourself.

All types of meditations are not the same. In this brief book we try to explain the distinction between Transcendental Meditation—which leads to transcendence—and contemplation and concentration, which do not produce the same physiological changes found during TM practice.

We hope that this book will answer some basic questions you might have regarding meditation, and will help clarify why the experience of Transcendental Consciousness should be a natural part of a vibrant and healthy life for both the individual and society.

Lincoln Norton
Fairfield Iowa, USA, March 1, 2016

Foreword

Foreword

Since its introduction in the United States in 1959, Transcendental Meditation has been the subject of extensive research. More than 600 studies, 380 of which have been published in leading peer-reviewed scientific journals, have demonstrated the profound and wide-ranging benefits of TM practice for mind, body, behavior, and society as a whole.

The basis of all these benefits, however, is the unique fourth state of consciousness experienced during TM practice, confirmed by research as completely different from waking, dreaming, and sleeping. TM practice effortlessly and automatically turns human attention within to experience and explore deeper levels of mind. This inward exploration of consciousness culminates in the experience of the simplest, most settled state of human awareness—a state of pure inner wakefulness or "pure consciousness"—accompanied by profound physiological rest that restores and revitalizes the mind and body.

As a scientist and educator, I am often asked how this process of transcending during TM—and how this experience of a field of "pure consciousness"—can be understood from the vantage point of modern science.

Let me answer that question by presenting a brief overview of our modern understanding of the universe—of reality—as seen from the perspective of quantum physics.

Science has discovered that nature has a hierarchical structure. During the course of the 20th century, physics sequentially uncovered deeper levels of physical reality—from the macroscopic to the microscopic, molecular, atomic, nuclear, and sub-nuclear levels of nature's functioning.

This inward exploration of deeper, progressively more unified levels of nature culminated in the recent discovery of completely unified field theories based on the superstring. These theories locate a single, universal, unified field of intelligence at the basis of all forms and phenomena in the Universe.

These deeper levels of physical reality are not only smaller—they are qualitatively, profoundly different. Each deeper level is governed by a unique set of physical laws; each possesses its own logic, its own natural language, its own mathematics. Entirely new physical theories and new mathematical frameworks had to be formulated to describe each new and deeper level of physical reality: theories that are known as quantum mechanics, quantum field theory, and unified field theory.

In a precisely parallel way, the human mind has been found to have a hierarchical structure. There is what is commonly referred to as the "surface level" of mind—the active thinking mind in which the awareness is directed outward through the macroscopic senses. But there are also deeper, quieter levels of mind, in which the awareness is more inwardly directed—the levels of "abstract thinking" and "fine feeling."

What Albert Einstein, Eugene Wigner, and many others have found most extraordinary is the remarkably precise parallel between this hierarchical structure of the human mind and the structure of physical nature. To quote Wigner (*a.k.a.* The Father of the Atomic Age): "The human mind fits nature—like a glove." This mysterious connection between mind and matter helps to explain why the human mind has the natural capacity to comprehend physical nature. As Einstein once said, "The most mysterious thing about the Universe is its comprehensibility by the mind."

Throughout human history—long before the birth of modern mathematics—there have been contemplative traditions and meditative methods for exploring deeper levels of mind, and by doing so, gaining a deeper comprehension of the Universe. The most ancient and highly developed of these meditative traditions—and the source of most other major traditions—is the Yogic science of meditation rooted in the Vedic tradition of ancient India.

The Yogic tradition developed systematic methodologies for drawing the attention deeply within to experience quieter, more expanded levels of awareness. This inward flow of the mind naturally culminates in the experience of the source of thought—pure consciousness—traditionally known as *samadhi.* In the language of physics, this maximally expanded state of awareness is the direct conscious experience/realization of the unified field—the fundamental unity at the basis of creation.

Modern physiological science has identified this state of samadhi as a fourth major state of human consciousness, physiologically and subjectively distinct from waking, dreaming, and deep sleep. Neurophysiologically, this experience is marked by the onset of global EEG coherence and increased alpha power, indicating peak orderliness of brain functioning and utilization of the total brain.

This fourth state of consciousness is universally accessible today through specific, highly developed technologies of consciousness derived from the Vedic tradition. Among these technologies, the Transcendental Meditation program and more advanced TM-Sidhi program of Maharishi Mahesh Yogi are the most extensively researched and widely practiced technologies in the world for accessing this fourth state—and thereby experiencing the many physiological, psychological, behavioral, and sociological benefits described in this book.

One key scientific point here is that when human awareness is maximally expanded—when human awareness opens to, and identifies itself with, the unbounded, universal unified field—then the nature and reach of this state of consciousness is non-localized and transpersonal. At that fundamental, spatially unbounded, unified level of reality, we are all, in essence, unified: we are all intimately and intricately connected as one universal field of consciousness—the unified field.

To state this succinctly, at its deepest, most expanded level, consciousness is a *field*. And field effects of consciousness—*i.e.*, long-range, society-wide effects of consciousness—are to be expected, and indeed, have been observed and reported in the extensive published research on collective consciousness mentioned in this book.

The precise neurological mechanisms that underlie the brain's ability to experientially access the unified field are rather sophisticated, and lie somewhat beyond the scope of this foreword. Briefly, it is increasingly accepted by researchers studying the neuroscience of consciousness that quantum mechanics plays a pivotal role in the phenomenon of consciousness—*i.e.*, that without quantum-mechanical effects in the brain, the intrinsic liveliness of experience we call "consciousness" would simply not exist.

Moreover, in a series of remarkable theoretical breakthroughs from string theory, it has been shown that wherever quantum mechanics is present (e.g., in brain processes associated with consciousness), the unified field is equally present; i.e., wherever quantum mechanics plays a role, string theory equally plays a role.

Therefore, phenomena previously understood as quantum-mechanical processes at the atomic or molecular scale can now be more accurately and properly viewed as string-theoretic phenomena—as phenomena of the unified field.

It follows directly that if consciousness has its biological roots in quantum-mechanical phenomena at the molecular-neuronal scale of the brain (as many neuroscientists now believe), then it is, in fact, more accurate to say that consciousness has its roots in the unified field—*i.e.,* that consciousness is a phenomenon of the unified field.

It is therefore not surprising, neurophysiologically, that consciousness, as it explores and gains intimate familiarity with its own fundamental nature during deep meditation, is also gaining intimate familiarity with—and direct contact with—the unified field.

In turn, as the research findings in this book will confirm, the direct experience of the unified field completely reorganizes brain activity, resulting in a unique state of orderliness of brain functioning called global EEG coherence. In this state, all areas of the brain—the left and right hemispheres, the frontal and occipital lobes, the temporal and parietal lobes of the brain—begin to function holistically, in concert, in a highly integrated way. Research further shows that EEG coherence is directly correlated with increased intelligence, IQ, creativity, learning ability, short-term and long-term memory, academic performance, moral reasoning, psychological stability, emotional maturity, alertness, and reaction time. Everything good about the brain depends on its orderly functioning. In addition, the profound physiological rest that accompanies this experience dissolves deep-rooted stress and restores physiological balance and health, leading to a host of positive outcomes for daily life and living.

I hope this brief presentation of insights from modern physics is helpful in explaining why Transcendental Meditation practice produces such profound and wide-ranging benefits for human life. This direct experience of the unified field transforms brain functioning, relieves deep-rooted stress, and revitalizes mind and body, leading to significantly greater success and enjoyment of life for anyone who practices the technique. TM practice is truly an educational breakthrough of the foremost magnitude.

John Hagelin, Ph.D.
International President, Global Union of Scientists for Peace

Introduction

Sometimes life is too busy. You can be lying in bed, trying to fall asleep, and virtually be climbing mountains in your mind—sleep is a million miles away. Or you might be reading a book and, at the bottom of the page, think to yourself, "I have no idea what I just read; my mind raced over the words!" Maybe it's not just your mind that's always racing. For most people, life can be so demanding that you sometimes wonder if you'll ever be free of the stress and exhaustion you live with on a daily basis.

Then there are times when you feel peace and happiness well up inside you. Perhaps you're on vacation enjoying nature—or maybe you're sitting with someone you care deeply about, feeling love flowing quietly between the two of you. It's probably safe to say that most of us would prefer to have this kind of experience over the constant stress of a busy life and a mind that never seems to be able to rest. But is there a way to experience peace and joy when you're not on vacation or in love?

The answer is yes. Transcendental Meditation (TM) is a technique that allows you to take an effortless break from the endless activity of your daily life, and experience the profound and restorative silence—the peace—that lies within each of us. It's a simple, natural mental technique that enables you to systematically experience the quiet levels of the mind (yes—they do exist!), reaching even the deepest part of the mind, where you'll find the source of your own inner happiness, intelligence, and creativity.

And here's the best part: When your short period of meditation is over, you bring that inner silence and creativity into your activity. A twenty-minute meditation twice a day dramatically reduces stress and strain in your entire physiology. Both your mind and body feel refreshed after meditating, and you have greater access to the deeper levels of intelligence and inspiration that reside in those quieter levels of the mind.

How is this possible, and what can you expect when you practice Transcendental Meditation? This book answers these frequently asked questions—and many more.

What You'll Find in This Book

The first two chapters are about the practice itself. Chapter 1, "What Is Transcendental Meditation?" describes TM—what it is and isn't. In this chapter, we'll look at the general benefits of TM, as well as how it differs from other kinds of meditation.

Chapter 2, "The Practice of Transcendental Meditation," examines the practical specifics of when to do it, for how long, etc.

Next, we'll get to some of the benefits of TM—which are extensively documented through scientific research. Chapter 3 discusses the effects of TM on health and aging, which include a whole range of positive influences on the body to keep us flexible and in good health as we age.

Chapter 4 is about long-term changes associated with the practice of Transcendental Meditation, which include the effects of TM on psychological well-being and the development of higher states of consciousness that have not been clearly understood until now.

And Chapter 5 looks at the effects of TM in education, offering profound implications for the improvement of our educational system as a whole.

In Chapter 6, "The Neurophysiology of Peace," we look at the connection between the practice of TM and its extraordinary effects on society.

Chapter 7 discusses the brain, consciousness, and enlightenment, exploring the unique capacity of TM to go far beyond everyday benefits and take the practitioner to what we call *enlightenment*, the ultimate state of self-realization, sought by all who are interested in the development of human potential. In this chapter, we'll also look at the loss and revival of the knowledge of enlightenment throughout the ages, and particularly how the re-enlivenment of the knowledge of TM represents one of the greatest gifts of our age.

TM is perfect for active people who feel they could be making greater use of their innate potential. It's for anyone looking for a way to relieve stress and restore and maintain good health. It's also for anyone who longs for a way to be at peace while meeting the demands of modern-day living. It's for parents who want to give their children a huge advantage at school—and in life. And it's for those who understand that who we *are* influences the world around us as much as (if not more than) what we *do*—so why not be the best we can be?

Whether you've just learned TM or are thinking about learning it, we're glad you've picked up this book because we believe TM will change your life for the better. So welcome! We look forward to meeting you along the way.

Chapter 1

What Is Transcendental Meditation?

Perhaps you've thought about learning how to meditate; you've heard about Transcendental Meditation, but you're not really sure what it is and whether it's for you. Or maybe you've just learned how to practice TM, and now that you have a little experience, you've got questions. Either way, *the point of this book is to answer your questions.*

In this chapter, we'll start with some basics: what TM is and what it isn't, how it works, who can practice it—and maybe a few things you haven't thought about asking yet. Your questions and our answers will help you understand the uniqueness of TM and how easy it is to learn and practice.

How does Transcendental Meditation work?

TM only takes twenty minutes, twice each day. You sit comfortably with your eyes closed. It involves no mood, belief, philosophy, or lifestyle. In fact, more than six million people of all ages, cultures, and religions have learned this effortless and effective technique of meditation. TM simply allows the mind to settle inward, through quieter levels of thought, until you experience the most silent and peaceful level of your own awareness. TM uses the natural tendency of the mind to spontaneously go to states of great happiness. Because of the intimate connection between the mind and body, as the mind settles to quieter, finer levels of thought, the body spontaneously achieves a state of profound rest, while brain activity becomes highly integrated (see Chapter 4). It is as if we have a switch in our nervous system that is automatically turned on during TM to produce this state of restful alertness. The result is that during TM you rejuvenate and revitalize the nervous system, and as a result you become more successful and fulfilled in activity.

Why do you call it "Transcendental" Meditation?

The word *transcend* means "to go beyond." Imagine that the mind is like an ocean, with the surface levels active and full of waves, and the depths very silent. Transcendental Meditation takes the awareness beyond the limitations of the active surface level of the mind—the sensory level of life—to deeper and subtler levels, until it reaches what could be called the simplest state of awareness: *pure consciousness.*

What is "pure consciousness" and why is it worth experiencing?

The transcendental state experienced during the practice of TM is called *pure consciousness* because it is awareness by itself, completely silent, without awareness of sounds, light, or any other sensory experience. Think about it: when you go about your normal life during your waking hours of consciousness, you're constantly thinking, feeling, and doing, as you're trying to *accomplish* something. But when you meditate with your eyes closed, your mind has a chance to settle down to quieter levels and actually have an experience of where your thoughts come from: the source of all thought, which is pure consciousness. Pure consciousness is consciousness *before* your feelings, thoughts, perceptions, and actions begin to take shape. It is the core reality that lies within all of us.

During TM practice, we experience pure consciousness at least briefly due to this natural settling down of the mind. Research shows that that this experience signifies a unique fourth state of consciousness, known as *Transcendental Consciousness*, that is completely distinct from the three ordinary states of consciousness we're used to: waking, dreaming, and sleeping. This fourth state has its own unique physiological characteristics, in which the body is experiencing deep rest while the mind is highly alert. Subjectively, no thoughts or sensations remain—only the experience of consciousness awake to itself. Physiologically, it is a state of restful alertness.

Can anybody learn TM?

TM is for people who lead active lives. Most people begin TM for practical reasons: they want better physical and mental health, increased energy, less anxiety and tension, more fulfilling relationships, greater clarity of thought, or more success and fulfillment.

Many individuals today experience the benefits of this highly effective meditation technique. We hear a lot about famous movie stars, business leaders, athletes, musicians, scientists, fashion models, and talk show hosts who all practice TM. But hundreds of thousands more —homemakers, teachers, bank clerks, farmers, small business persons, students of all ages, veterans, and people from every imaginable walk of life—are quietly and effortlessly practicing the TM program, benefiting from the proven release of stress and increasing their success and happiness at work and at home.

What benefits can I expect if I practice TM?

Extensive research has documented the effectiveness of TM in improving both physical and mental health. TM helps every area of life by removing stress from your nervous system, which allows your mind and body to function more effectively. Stress has been called "the black plague" of our generation, and stress comes from any kind of overloading of the nervous system. This overloading can come from different sources, and it happens even though we all know that when we're well rested, we're far more creative and productive than when we're tired or stressed.

Unfortunately, the rest we get during sleep is not enough to remove a lifetime of deep stress. During Transcendental Meditation, however, the profound state of rest gained by the physiology begins to dissolve these accumulated stresses. (1). As a result, we have more energy, our mental abilities become sharper, our health improves, our emotions become balanced, and we become happier and more effective in daily life.

What research, if any, has been done on TM?

More than 600 studies at more than 200 research institutes and universities have been conducted on the Transcendental Meditation program, and over 380 of those studies have been published in peer-reviewed journals. "Peer-reviewed" means that scientists with qualifications and competencies similar to those of the study authors have evaluated the work. These methods are the gold standard of science, employed to maintain the highest standards of quality and credibility.

When a person experiences transcending, his or her physiology reaches a very deep state of rest—yet at the same time, the person's mind is completely clear and alert. The principal finding of scientific research on Transcendental Meditation is, as we said earlier, that it provides the experience of a fourth major state of consciousness: Transcendental Consciousness.

What makes TM different from other forms of meditation?

The practices of Zen, Compassion Meditation, Quigong, Diamond Way Buddhism, Zazen, Kriya Yoga, and the more recent practices of Mindfulness and Mindfulness-Based Stress Reduction (MBSR) are different from Transcendental Meditation. Scientists Dr. Fred Travis and Dr. Jonathan Shear have published a paper in which they identify three major categories of "meditation" out of more than a hundred different practices (2). These three are summarized as follows:

Focused attention: The first type of practice can be described as *concentration meditation,* since in this case, the practitioner puts his or her attention intently on something (it might be a word, an emotion, a candle flame, etc.). The changes in the brain are in the gamma range (20–50 Hz), which is known to be associated with this type of focused activity. Some forms of Zen, Compassion Meditation, Quigong, and Diamond Way Buddhism are in this category.

Open monitoring: This second of type of practice can be described as *contemplation meditation.* In this process, the practitioner watches himself or herself do something, such as paying attention to thoughts or the breath. This category includes Zazen, Kriya Yoga, and more recently developed versions of meditation like Mindfulness. The changes in the brain from these meditations are in the theta range (4–8 Hz), known to be associated with imagination and creativity.

Automatic self-transcending: This third type of practice can be described as *transcending meditation.* In this practice there is no trying, no concentration, and no contemplation—only effortless transcending. The changes in the brain are in the alpha 1 range (8–10 Hz) and are correlated with an eyes-closed, relaxed state of restful alertness. Transcendental Meditation is this third type of meditation—which, as you will discover, produces numerous physical and psychological benefits in activity.

Is it possible to fail the TM course?

Some people think they can't meditate because their minds are too active; others think they can't do it because it will be too hard. TM uses the nature of the mind to go to fields of greater happiness—to go within. No "trying" is involved. If you try, your mind remains on the surface and cannot dive deep. Transcendence is a real experience that isn't based on a mood or emotion.

The fact is that nobody can fail the TM course! Transcendental Meditation is for everyone. TM, as we said, involves effortless transcending as the natural outcome of the mind's inherent tendency to move toward greater charm—which is why nobody can fail. TM has been taught to millions of people around the world. Anyone from any educational background—or no educational background—can easily learn TM.

Is TM a religious practice?

No. TM comes from the Vedic tradition of India, which predates Hinduism, but it's not exclusive to any culture, religion, or country. It's not religious any more than the yoga classes offered by your local YMCA are religious. India is the home of this ancient knowledge, but this doesn't mean that TM is either Indian or Hindu. Sir Isaac Newton discovered gravity, but gravity is certainly neither British nor Christian. TM is a universal technique that makes use of the natural ability of the mind to transcend; the nervous system settles down correspondingly into a state that supports this subjective experience of transcendence. It's not even necessary for you to believe that TM will work in order for you to experience its benefits!

Where does TM come from?

Maharishi Mahesh Yogi was the founder of the Transcendental Meditation technique and its advanced programs. Maharishi's genius was his rediscovery of certain time-tested procedures for the development of consciousness in active people. Maharishi was also responsible for encouraging researchers at leading universities around the world to conduct physiological, psychological, and sociological studies on the effects of the TM program (the TM "program" refers to both the TM technique and other advanced techniques we'll mention later).

Maharishi explains that the technique of effortless transcending in TM is many thousands of years old and was passed on to him by his teacher, Brahmananda Saraswati—or Guru Dev, as Maharishi often referred to him. Renowned throughout India for his vast knowledge and understanding of the ancient Vedic tradition, Guru Dev occupied the seat of Shankaracharya of northern India, a position vacant for over 150 years until a figure of his spiritual stature could at last do it justice. We acknowledge him as being in the direct line of expert teachers who have preserved and passed down this profound knowledge.

When you embark on learning TM, there is a short nonreligious ceremony to honor the tradition of knowledge from which TM comes. As the student, you are simply a witness to the ceremony. This part of the teaching procedure reminds the teacher that he or she did not originate this meditation— that it comes from an ancient and renowned tradition. Also, when the teacher comes from the busy modern world, this procedure helps to settle his or her mind in preparation for teaching.

Why does TM require personal instruction?

While the experience of transcending can be verbally described (and there have been numerous literary descriptions of it over the centuries), it's an experience that depends upon a very specific and delicate state of the nervous system. It cannot properly be learned from books but must be taught through the personal instruction of a thoroughly trained teacher. Among other things, correct instruction helps the meditator avoid any "trying," straining, or expectation, all of which, according to Maharishi, hold the mind on the gross level and prevent the experience of more delicate and subtle levels of the thinking process.

How do I learn TM?

TM is taught in seven steps, normally done within a week's time according to your schedule. Most of the steps take one to two hours (though some are shorter). There are also brief but important follow-up meetings ten days after you learn the practice and then once a month for the first three months after your TM course. The seven steps are outlined at the back of this book. All of these meetings are included in your course fee, as is lifelong support for your meditation program, including personal checking, advanced meetings, and other special events. The course fee is different for every country, and further details are given in the appendices.

Chapter 2

The Practice of Transcendental Meditation

Now that you know what makes TM different from other forms of meditation and how easy it is to learn and practice, let's look at some specifics of the practice.

What makes this technique "natural"? What are the logistics—how long, how often, and at what time of day do you meditate? And is it possible that your meditation practice can affect those around you? These are just a few of the questions we'll answer in this chapter about the practice of TM.

Why is the process of transcending so effortless with TM?

Many systems of meditation teach that the tendency of the mind is to wander and that in order to experience quieter levels of consciousness, the mind must be disciplined or controlled through long practice. Maharishi has corrected this misunderstanding, explaining that the natural tendency of the mind is not to wander aimlessly or jump around like a monkey but rather to move in the direction of experiences that bring us greater happiness and enjoyment—just as a honeybee moves naturally toward a flower. Maharishi has also pointed out that increasingly quiet and more refined levels of thinking are progressively more enjoyable. And since the TM technique makes use of the mind's inherent tendency to move toward greater enjoyment, we only need to know how to begin the TM technique correctly in order for the attention to be spontaneously drawn inward. However, while this process of transcending is completely easy, effortless, and natural, it is also delicate. Without proper instruction and "checking" by a qualified TM teacher, misunderstandings and straining may arise, leaving the meditator without the full benefits of the practice.

Can anyone transcend through TM?

Yes! A new TM practitioner is just as capable of transcending as a long-term meditator. This is supported not only by the direct experience of new meditators but also by scientific research showing that the EEG characteristics of transcending are similar in both new and long-term meditators (3). The difference seen in long-term meditators is not in the ability to transcend but rather in activity. Over time, TM practice dissolves a great deal of stress, and therefore long-term meditators have naturally stabilized a higher level of EEG coherence in activity, which is correlated with higher levels of intelligence, creativity, and learning ability, leading to greater effectiveness and more fulfillment in daily life (4). (See Chapter 4 for more on the long-term benefits of TM.)

As described in Chapter 1, TM is different from other forms of meditation. It doesn't involve any form of concentration, contemplation, or mindfulness, in which some effort may be involved. Instead, it's an effortless technique that produces positive results from the first time it is practiced. Because it's effortless, easy, and natural, nobody fails to transcend—and with the first experiences of transcendence, everyone begins to enjoy benefits. Only if effort creeps into the TM practice may it start to become difficult or uncomfortable—and to guard against this possibility, Maharishi also introduced a simple checking procedure that can restore effortlessness in TM practice very quickly so that benefits in daily life continue to grow.

What is the role of the mantra in TM practice?

In TM practice, the mantra is the vehicle for the transcending process. When you learn TM, you'll learn your mantra and how to use it properly to experience effortless transcending. The mantra's value is as sound—no meaning is associated with it, because meaning tends to hold the mind on the surface level of thinking, rather than allowing the mind to transcend to the source of thought.

The mantras used in the TM program come from the ancient Vedic tradition of India and are chosen in order to produce the greatest life-supporting and harmonious influence for each meditator. This principle is especially important as you experience finer levels of thinking, which are more powerful. The validation of the effectiveness of the TM mantras in enabling the mind to transcend is based on the many thousands of years of experience of the teachers of this tradition. It is also confirmed by the increased integration of brain functioning during TM practice, which is correlated with many psychological and behavioral improvements.

Does it take willpower or discipline to meditate?

Not with TM practice. The idea that meditation requires willpower or discipline comes from the misunderstanding that meditation is difficult and involves control, as may be the case with other practices. The TM practice is natural, effortless, and enjoyable. The only thing you need to do is to learn the TM technique—and then simply make TM part of your daily routine. One meditator said, "While it's true that I have not missed a meditation in thirty years, it's also true that I haven't missed breakfast in thirty years, so it's not a question of willpower." We are *naturally motivated* to continue because TM produces so many benefits.

How often should I meditate and for how long?

TM is practiced for only about twenty minutes each morning and evening, while sitting comfortably with the eyes closed, and it can therefore easily be incorporated into even a very demanding life. By allowing us to dive deep within and transcend repeatedly, TM practice infuses the mind with greater creativity and energy, which helps to make us more effective and successful in all our daily activities. In the evening, when we're tired and in need of rest, twenty minutes of meditation helps to restore our mind and body and prepares us for our evening activity.

Can I meditate more than twice a day?

Meditating twice a day is the most effective program for an active person. Maharishi used a simple analogy to explain this. In the villages of India, cloth is often colored by placing it in a vat of dye and then spreading it in the sun to fade. In the hot sun, the cloth naturally begins to fade back to its original color, so it is again placed in the dye for a short time and put back in the sun to fade. By alternating the cloth's exposure to the dye and the sun, the color becomes fixed. For this purpose, it's of no benefit to leave the cloth in the dye for a longer period of time, nor does it help to leave it longer in the sun.

Consequently, for the quickest infusion of the benefits of TM practice into daily life, we meditate for twenty minutes in the morning and then engage in normal activity during the day; and then at the end of the day, when our "batteries" start to wear down, we again meditate to prepare for our evening activity. Rest and activity are both necessary in order to refine the nervous system to be more effective in its functioning. By alternating the experience of pure consciousness and normal activity in this way, we culture the nervous system to maintain our experience of pure consciousness—the source of creative intelligence—at all times. Maharishi spoke of this outcome as living 200 percent of life—100 percent of inner life and 100 percent outer life.

Can I meditate just before bed?

TM gives us energy as a preparation for activity. To increase your energy right before sleep is not a great idea because it's likely to keep you awake.

Can I meditate more when I feel I need it?

TM isn't meant to be a Band-Aid for specific problems, but there are a few exceptions. If you are seriously ill in bed or in the hospital, for example, additional TM practice can help you gain deeper rest and heal more quickly. Also, if you are a student, you might meditate for a few minutes before an exam to help clear your mind. Be sure to check with your TM teacher and ask when it might be appropriate to add an occasional meditation.

Are there any other techniques I can learn after TM?

There are a number of advanced TM programs; however, TM is always the core technique, and it will continue to benefit your life whether you choose to take an advanced program or not. Maharishi described advanced techniques as "fertilizers" that help stabilize the experience of pure consciousness and accelerate the growth to higher states of consciousness (See Chapter 4). You can speak with a TM teacher to find out more about these advanced programs.

Chapter 3

The Effects of Transcendental Meditation
on Health and Aging

One of the most significant areas of benefit that separates TM from other forms of meditation is its extraordinary effects on health and aging. As mentioned earlier, 380 scientific studies have substantiated TM-related improvements in every aspect of mental and physical health.

What illnesses and physical conditions can be improved by the practice of TM? Can it lower your high blood pressure? Can it help PTSD? Can it make you younger? These important questions are addressed in this chapter.

How does TM affect health?

We have explained that the mind settles down during TM and experiences finer, quieter levels of thinking. But mind and body are intimately connected. You know from your own experience that when you're exhausted from too much mental work, your body also feels tired. And when you haven't gotten enough sleep, it's difficult to be alert, think clearly, and make decisions easily. This mind/body connection allows for one of the most profound aspects of TM: when your mind settles down during the practice, your body also naturally settles down into a deeply restful state.

This deep rest is responsible for both the release of stress and the restoration of health. Hundreds of studies documenting the health benefits of TM have been conducted at such leading institutions as Harvard and Yale Medical Schools and published in prestigious medical journals. The US National Institutes of Health have awarded $25 million to study the effects of TM on health, particularly on heart disease, the number-one killer in the USA.

How does TM affect heart disease?

A number of studies have shown that TM has a positive impact on heart disease. One of the most significant studies found that African Americans with heart disease who practiced the TM technique regularly were 48 percent less likely to have a heart attack or stroke, or to die from other causes, as compared with African Americans who attended a health education class for more than five years. It is particularly interesting to note that researchers who conducted the study at the Medical College of Wisconsin in Milwaukee reported that the more regularly the patients meditated, the longer their term of survival (5).

What are the effects of TM on high blood pressure?

A number of important studies have shown that TM reduces high blood pressure. A scientific statement from the American Heart Association concluded, "The Transcendental Meditation technique is the only meditation practice that has been shown to lower blood pressure" (6).

Other quotes from the same statement include the following:

> "Because of many negative studies or mixed results and a paucity of available trials, all other meditation techniques (including MBSR) received a 'Class III, no benefit, Level of Evidence C' recommendation. Thus, other meditation techniques are not recommended in clinical practice to lower BP at this time."

> "Transcendental Meditation practice is recommended for consideration in treatment plans for all individuals with blood pressure > 120/80 mm Hg."

> "Lower blood pressure through Transcendental Meditation practice is also associated with substantially reduced rates of death, heart attack, and stroke."

Can TM reduce other risk factors that influence heart disease?

Yes. Research has shown that TM practice reduces cholesterol levels and tobacco use (7), and it also helps to improve certain at-risk conditions, such as diabetes and obesity (see next section). In addition, TM lowers or eliminates stress, which exacerbates heart disease and many other disorders. Studies show that meditators exhibit an improved ability to adapt to stressful situations and a marked decrease in levels of plasma cortisol, commonly known as the "stress hormone"(8).

What about diabetes?

A critical factor in recovering from diabetes is insulin resistance. A randomized clinical trial, funded by the National Institutes of Health, revealed significant improvements in TM subjects (as compared with a control group) in the levels of insulin resistance in those with coronary heart disease (9).

Approximately 70 percent of all American Indians suffer from diabetes, and TM has been introduced in several American Indian reservations and schools. Preliminary research shows that TM significantly decreases diabetes, reduces stress, and normalizes high blood pressure in this population. Research also shows improved self-confidence, positivity, and happiness, with increases in grade-point average and graduation rates among American Indian students (10).

Can TM improve other areas of health?

Research results in other areas of health show improvements in such conditions as asthma, insomnia, pain, alcohol and drug abuse, and mental health (11). A recent random-ized controlled trial of 130 older women with breast cancer showed that in every case, Transcendental Meditation im-proved their quality of life (12).

Can TM reduce medical costs?

In terms of health care costs, several important studies have revealed the significant effects of TM. In a five-year study on some two thousand individuals, Dr. David Orme-Johnson showed that meditators use medical and surgical health care services approximately one-half as often as do other insur-ance users. This study was conducted in cooperation with Blue Cross–Blue Shield and controlled for other factors that might affect health care use, such as cost sharing, age, gender, geographic distribution, and profession. The TM subjects also showed a far lower rate of increase in health care utiliza-tion with increasing age (13).

In Québec, Canada, Dr. Robert Herron and coworkers compared the changes in physician costs for TM practitioners with those of non-practitioners over a five-year period. This study was particularly reliable because the Canadian govern-ment was able to track health care costs closely for both the meditators and the control group, due to Canada's national health care system. After the first year, the TM group's health care costs decreased 11 percent, and after five years, their cumulative cost reduction was 28 percent. The TM patients required fewer referrals, resulting in lower medical expenses for things such as tests, prescription drugs, hospitalization, surgery, and other treatments (14).

What about PTSD?

Over half a million US troops deployed since 2001 suffer from PTSD. Yet due to ineffective treatments and a lack of government resources, less than 20 percent of these military personnel and veterans will receive adequate care. It's estimated that at least half of those with PTSD will receive no care at all and are at great risk for violent and self-destructive behavior.

Key findings on the effects of TM on PTSD include a 40–55 percent reduction in the symptoms of PTSD and depression, a 42 percent decrease in insomnia, and a 30 percent improvement in satisfaction with the individual's quality of life. The physiological and psychological improvements gained during the regular practice of TM provide a safe and effective way to relieve the debilitating effects of PTSD. TM also helps to restore resilience in both soldiers on active duty and veterans returning home. TM has been introduced into a number of military institutions in the United States and around the world. At the time of this writing, a well-controlled research study funded by the US Department of Defense is being conducted on a large population of veterans (15).

How can one simple mental technique bring about all these changes?

Earlier in this chapter, we said that the mind and body are intimately connected. Every single experience we have changes the brain. The experience of transcending during TM changes the activity of the brain in a way that enables us to experience higher states of consciousness and greater success and fulfillment.

Recent research has revealed that TM practice changes not only the brain but also the most fundamental level of the physiology: the expression of genes in DNA. One study shows that TM affects the expression of over seventy genes; another shows that it increases the expression of a particular gene that could help reverse the aging process (16). Scientists have only started to unravel how it is that by changing the expression of specific genes, TM can create so many benefits for health and aging.

How does TM affect aging?

Aging may be inevitable, but the rate at which each person ages is not fixed. Why and how our bodies age is still largely a mystery, although we're learning more each year. Scientists maintain, however, that chronological age has little bearing on biological age.

Aging is the inevitable decline in the body's resiliency, which ultimately leads to dwindling mental and physical power. But which affects us more—our genes or our lifestyles? Although the cells we received from our parents strongly affect our aging process, they are not the only factor.

Aging is complicated, and it's often difficult to distinguish between changes that are the result of time and those that come with medical conditions, such as arthritis and heart disease. But lifestyle is key. We often operate at high speed day after day, without ever really getting deep rest. This results in constant wear and tear. By practicing TM to give your body the deep rest it needs to rejuvenate on a daily basis, you automatically give yourself an advantage few people have.

Has there been research on TM and aging?

Many studies have documented how TM can slow and even reverse the aging process (17). One study shows that long-term TM meditators have a biological age roughly twelve years younger than their non-meditating counterparts. And we've already discussed numerous studies showing that TM improves many aspects of health and the quality of life (18).

Researchers at Harvard University studied the effects of TM on mental health, behavioral flexibility, blood pressure, and longevity in residents of homes for the elderly. The subjects were randomly assigned to either a no-treatment group or one of three treatment programs: the TM program, mindfulness training, or a relaxation program. All three groups were initially similar on pretest measures and in expectancy of benefits, yet after a three-month experimental period, the TM group had significant improvements in cognitive functioning and blood pressure as compared to the control groups. Also, the TM subjects reported feeling more absorbed during their practice and better and more relaxed immediately afterward than did the mindfulness or the relaxation subjects. Overall, more TM subjects found their practice to be personally valuable than did member of either of the control groups (19).

The most striking finding was that TM practice reversing not only age-related declines in overall health, but also directly enhanced longevity. All members of the TM group were still alive three years after the program began, in contrast to about only half of the members of the control groups. Research on the Transcendental Meditation program clearly shows that growing old no longer needs to signify a loss in the quality of life; rather, it can be an opportunity for further development.

Chapter 4

Long-Term Changes Associated with
Regular Transcendental Meditation Practice

You now know what TM can do for you in the short term—even immediately. Most people report feeling very relaxed even at their first instructional session, and the benefits begin to be felt right away.

But what about long-term effects? We're glad you asked: TM has been around long enough that there are now thousands of meditators who have been practicing TM for forty or more years. They can attest to the cumulative effects of their practice, which can also be scientifically measured. And again, extensive research demonstrates the ongoing health benefits of practicing TM over time.

There's more: In Chapter 2, we spoke briefly about higher states of consciousness. We will now go into greater detail about the exalted states of human potential that are possible through the long-term practice of TM.

What are some of the long-term changes that come with the practice of TM?

The effects of twice-daily practice of TM have been proven to be cumulative. As mentioned earlier, hundreds of studies document the long-term benefits of daily meditation. TM practice affects gene expression, improves blood pressure, reduces cardiovascular disease, and assists in all areas of health. Long-term changes in brain functioning have also been correlated with increased creativity, intelligence, and learning ability.

One important psychological study on TM shows a significant decrease in levels of anxiety in TM practitioners as compared to subjects practicing other relaxation techniques (20). Psychological studies show that long-term TM practice decreases neuroticism, depression, and aggression, and increases self-esteem, moral reasoning, and self-actualization (21). Studies in a variety of work and business settings show increased productivity and efficiency (22).

What about long-term effects in terms of higher states of consciousness?

Maharishi described seven states of consciousness, three of which are generally considered "normal": the waking state, the dreaming state, and the sleeping state. According to the

Vedic tradition, however, there are four other, *higher* states of consciousness that are possible to experience. The first of these is called Transcendental Consciousness, in which we experience the state of pure consciousness described in Chapter 1. It is experienced as a state of restful alertness. It is distinctly different from waking, dreaming, and sleeping and is the basis for development of the other higher states. With the regular practice of TM, a person's mind and body eventually become free from stress, and this results in a shift in the functioning of the nervous system so that it can support higher states of consciousness.

Studies have documented the unique set of physiological and biochemical characteristics of this fourth state of consciousness that occurs during TM practice (23). The brain shows patterns of wakeful orderliness—*global EEG coherence*—indicating improved integration and communication among different parts of the brain. At the same time, the body enters a very deep state of rest, characterized by a decrease in certain autonomic, metabolic, biochemical, and hormonal functions.

Over time, the regular experience of the fourth state of consciousness begins to yield other higher states.

What are these other higher states?

The fifth state is called Cosmic Consciousness, which is traditionally described as the coexistence of pure consciousness along with waking, dreaming, and sleeping states. For example, in the fifth state, even when a person is sleeping, he or she continues to enjoy the underlying blissful experience of the deep, peaceful silence of pure consciousness.

Further refinement of neurophysiological functioning results in two other higher states, which are known as *Refined Cosmic Consciousness* and *Unity Consciousness*. The ancient Vedic literature of India describes the state of Refined Cosmic Consciousness as a state in which pure consciousness is maintained along with the ability to perceive the full range of creation, from its surface values to its deepest level—an experience that gives rise to profound appreciation and love for the perfection and beauty of nature. Refined Cosmic Consciousness evolves naturally in those who have achieved Cosmic Consciousness. In the seventh state, Unity Consciousness, everything is experienced in terms of the unboundedness of one's Self—the whole creation is cognized in terms of its limitless, infinite reality, which is nothing other than the reality of one's own infinite Self.

Is there scientific research to document the development of these states?

Several researchers have studied the EEG patterns of advanced TM meditators who reported the experience of pure consciousness throughout their sleeping, dreaming, and waking states—the subjective experience of Cosmic Consciousness (24). In the sleep study, these subjects showed a unique brainwave pattern, composed of two types of brain waves: the normal EEG patterns of deep sleep (delta waves) with superimposed EEG patterns of restful alertness (alpha waves). These findings provide an objective correlate for the coexistence of sleep state and pure consciousness experienced by these TM practitioners.

In studies on subjects experiencing pure consciousness during the waking state, one researcher developed a unique combination of EEG measures to assess the growth of higher states of consciousness. The researchers called this system of measures the Brain Integration Scale (BIS). The BIS is composed of three measures: EEG alpha coherence, EEG alpha power, and Contingent Negative Variation (CNV). Taken together, the BIS scores clearly show the cumulative long-term effects of TM practice and may be used to chart the growth of higher states of consciousness. Interestingly, this measure has also been used to study brain functioning in successful athletes, managers, and musicians, with the conclusion that higher BIS scores correlate with greater efficiency, effectiveness, and success in daily life (25).

Can anyone achieve higher states of consciousness?

Anyone with a functional human nervous system may achieve higher states of consciousness, according to Maharishi. The TM technique facilitates this process by providing the regular experience of transcending, resulting in a gradual refinement of neurophysiological functioning and an increase in mental potential. This process may be further accelerated with advanced TM techniques.

What is the relationship between TM and "self-actualization"?

One well-known Western psychologist, Abraham Maslow, described people who seek higher states of consciousness as "transcending self-actualizers." He writes about the self-actualizing man as not being an ordinary man with something added, but rather as the ordinary man with nothing taken away. Abraham Maslow's description of self-actualization has a number of similarities to descriptions of the growth of higher states of consciousness, which comes about naturally as the result of practicing TM.

According to Maslow, there are two basic types of individuals: those who are *deficiency motivated* and those who are *growth motivated.* Maslow explained that if a person is deficiency motivated, he or she is able to perceive and cognize the world only in a manner organized by his or her needs. On the other hand, the growth-motivated person perceives and experiences different values in the world. According to Maslow, such individuals have already sufficiently gratified their basic needs for safety, belongingness, love, respect, and self-esteem, and they are motivated further by a desire for "self-actualization." Among the values perceived and experienced by this kind of individual are wholeness, unity, completeness, playfulness, honesty, self-sufficiency, and integration. Such values, according to Maslow, are often present in what he called *peak experiences* or *transcendent experiences.* Maslow considered that the absence of these experiences indicated a lesser state of human development, in which we are not fully integrated.

Maslow identified two kinds of self-actualizing people: those "with little or no experience of transcendence, and those in whom transcendent experience was important— even central." Maslow felt that "transcending self-actualizers" were, among other things, more inclined to be responsive to beauty, more holistic in their perception of the world, more lovable and inspiring, more apt to be innovators, more likely to have strong self-knowledge, more open and humble, and more integrated and self-confident. All of these characteristics, as delineated by Maslow, are remarkably parallel to the characteristics traditionally recognized in individuals living higher states of consciousness, as described by Maharishi and by TM meditators around the globe.

Chapter 5

The Effects of Transcendental Meditation in Education

It's one thing to experience personal benefits through the practice of TM. But the introduction of TM into schools around the world is demonstrating the extraordinary impact that this meditation technique can have on educational systems and children at risk—as well as on society as a whole.

In this chapter, we'll share examples of what happens to students in schools where TM has been implemented as an integrated part of the curriculum. The results are astonishing.

Is there any research showing that TM is useful in education?

Numerous studies show that TM improves different aspects of student life—including increased academic performance; reduced anxiety; increased energy level; and improved self-esteem, tolerance, creativity, and intelligence. One study conducted on college students showed that over a two-year period, the IQ of the TM subjects increased significantly as compared to that of the control group—even though the general understanding has been that IQ does not change after age twenty (26).

Are there examples of how TM has improved entire schools?

The TM technique has been learned by students in hundreds of schools in the United States and other countries, with outstanding results. For example, with sponsorship from the David Lynch Foundation, over 7,000 inner-city children in San Francisco have learned the TM program in the context of school-wide "Quiet Time" programs. During Quiet Time, both faculty and students meditate for about ten minutes in the morning and ten minutes in the afternoon as part of the school day.

The first school to get involved in San Francisco was a "fight school," with suspensions nearly double the district average for middle schools. The high levels of student and faculty stress were negatively impacting student grades and attendance and contributing to high faculty turnover. TM was introduced into the school in the spring of 2007, resulting in a dramatic turnaround. In the first semester of the program, suspensions in the two grades that learned TM dropped 45% compared with the grade that didn't. After three years, schoolwide suspensions were half of the district average. In addition, schoolwide GPA improved, attendance increased, the percentage of students going to the top academic high school quintupled, and teacher turnover dropped sharply. In 2008, the school principal was selected National Middle School Principal of the Year. Published research on the effects of introducing TM in schools has found increases in graduation rates, standardized test scores, student attendance, and physical health, as well as reductions in suspensions, student anxiety and stress, and teacher burnout (27).

Another remarkable example of TM in education comes from the Fletcher Johnson Education Center, a low-income charter school with 1500 students in Washington, DC. The TM program was introduced there by Dr. George Rutherford, a top educator in the Washington, DC, area for over thirty-five years. More than 150 students and 85 percent of Dr. Rutherford's staff learned the TM technique as part of their Quiet Time program. The results were dramatic, including reductions in fighting and violence and improvements in both test scores and student-teacher interactions. In most cases, the teachers and the parents also started to practice TM, and this proved enormously helpful to the families.

The TM program was also introduced at Nataki Talibah Schoolhouse, a charter school in downtown Detroit, Michigan. In a study conducted by researchers at the University of Michigan, the meditating children showed significantly more positive emotions, positive mood states, and greater emotional adaptability than their non-meditating peers.

Meditating children also had higher self-esteem, more positive experiences of well-being, improved ability to manage stress, and better interpersonal skills—with less verbal aggression, anxiety, and loneliness (28).

The improvements seen in Detroit have been replicated in other schools wherever TM has been introduced. Teachers comment that classes become more settled, there is greater mutual respect, and students are more eager to learn and to perform better.

The Chelsea School, a private school in Silver Spring, MD, offered the TM program to children in grades 5 through 12 who had attention deficit-hyperactivity disorder (ADHD). Researchers showed that the TM practice could be learned and successfully practiced by children with ADHD—resulting in less stress, anxiety, and stress-related ADHD symptoms, as well as significant improvements in brain functioning—within three months (29).

What is the David Lynch Foundation and its relationship with TM?

David Lynch is a highly respected film director and artist who began to practice the TM technique over thirty-five years ago. Because of the benefits he experienced, he set up a foundation to bring these same benefits to at-risk populations, both in the United States and abroad.

The David Lynch Foundation has brought Transcendental Meditation to over half a million school children in the United States, Brazil, Peru, Bolivia, Vietnam, Nepal, Northern Ireland, Ghana, Kenya, Uganda, South Africa, and Israel. In addition, it has provided TM practice to veterans, female victims of domestic violence and abuse, soldiers and refugees suffering from PTSD, prisoners, the homeless, and American Indians—all with positive results. For details about the research on these and ongoing projects, see DavidLynch-Foundation.org.

Why is TM so effective for students?

By incorporating the TM technique into his or her daily routine, each student can develop greater mental potential through the progressive refinement of brain functioning. In this way, TM expands the "container of knowledge," rather than trying to stuff it with more and more information. Complete education, therefore, involves the systematic development of the brain, along with the purification and refinement of the entire physiology.

What does education have to do with physiology?

We don't normally think of education as a physiological experience—but it is. As a result of our educational experiences, we acquire a particular style or pattern of brain functioning. Unfortunately, the style generally ingrained by modern education tends to be a highly imbalanced learning pattern, in which students actually learn to overtax and stress themselves. The result is clearly seen in the prevalence of stress-related diseases, both mental and physical. It is as if we are literally conditioning our children to adopt a style of physiological functioning that forces them to consume large quantities of medication, such as antidepressants or anti-anxiety drugs, in order to cope with the stresses of life. Almost everyone today must deal with extraordinary social pressures that reflect the breakdown of life-supporting values within our families, communities, and society, so there is a critical need for education programs that can teach students how to unfold their full creative potential. The TM technique offers exactly this opportunity to education.

A number of studies have shown the effects of TM on students at different universities. In a well-controlled study at American University in Washington, DC, for example, researchers reported that students practicing TM for only three months showed decreased stress, anxiety, and depression and increased vitality, emotional and behavioral coping, creativity, and intelligence, as compared to control subjects (30).

Are there any schools or universities founded by Maharishi?

Maharishi founded many schools and universities all around the world. In the United States, Maharishi founded the Maharishi School of the Age of Enlightenment (K through 12) and Maharishi University of Management in Fairfield, Iowa. Students from the Maharishi School have earned the highest recognition in everything from science fairs to tennis, from theater to National Merit Scholarships. Maharishi University of Management is accredited to the doctoral level. Research on students at these institutions shows increased practical intelligence, self-development, and happiness, as well as improvements in brain functioning and physical and emotional health (31).

Chapter 6

The Neurophysiology of Peace

It's easy to see how TM practice can help foster individual peace. But it's often the case that individuals begin TM for the *express purpose of creating world peace*. Many consider their personal practice the greatest contribution they can make to our planet. And research shows that large groups of TM practitioners meditating together produce an extraordinary influence on the environment—another compelling example of TM's potential to affect society. .

Let's consider the connection between TM and peace, and the concept of *collective consciousness*.

How can there be any connection between the practice of TM and societal peace?

We are not just isolated individuals. We know that if one member of a family is unhappy or stressed, it affects the good feelings and happiness of the whole family. This is also true for a community and even a nation. As individuals, we influence and contribute to these different levels of collective consciousness—local, national, and global—and they in turn affect us.

As described by Dr. John Hagelin in the Foreword, recently discovered unified field theories of modern physics have located a single, universal, unified field of intelligence at the basis of all forms and phenomena in the universe. Scientists have postulated that when individuals transcend during TM practice, they gain access to this unified field—an experience that transforms the functioning of body and mind. *By gaining access to the unified field, which underlies and connects everything, they create an influence of coherence on that level that propagates throughout the collective consciousness of society and has a positive influence on the behavior of all the individuals in that society.* It's like throwing a rock into a pond: the waves go out in all directions, influencing the whole pond. In the same way, we influence those around us, whether we're aware of it or not. When we increase our own sense of inner calm and peace, that is what we radiate to the world around us.

What is the significance of the unified field of consciousness?

We've all had experiences, however ephemeral, of feeling something greater than our individual existence and activities—perhaps that we are one with nature or with another person. These experiences make sense today because we now know from science that there is a deep level of nature in which everything and everyone is connected. Einstein predicted that scientists would discover this underlying unified field and develop a "theory of everything"—and modern physics is developing reliable and testable theories that there is indeed one unified field of all matter and energy.

According to Maharishi Mahesh Yogi, founder of the TM technique, this unified field of matter and energy at the basis of the physical universe is the same as the unified field of pure consciousness experienced during the practice of TM. Each of us is part of nature, and inside all of us is that same unified field. This is the source of our awareness—our waking consciousness and all our unconscious thoughts, which arise until we become conscious of them as specific thoughts on the "surface" or active level of our mind. The unified field is the source of everything, and it enables our individual awareness—and consequently our individual thinking and action—to be connected with all of nature around us.

When did scientists first study the effects of TM on society?

In 1960, Maharishi Mahesh Yogi predicted that *one percent of a population practicing the Transcendental Meditation technique would produce measurable improvements in the quality of life for the whole population.* This phenomenon was first studied in 1974 and was referred to as the "Maharishi Effect." In 1976, Maharishi brought out several advanced programs derived from the Vedic tradition, which greatly enhanced the Maharishi Effect. Scientists found that when even the *square root of one percent* of any population practices these programs in a group, there is a measurable marked reduction in violence and an improvement in the quality of life.

Has there been any research to prove that TM can create peace in the world?

Over fifty studies, as we mentioned in Chapter 2, document the beneficial effects of the practice of TM and its advanced programs on reducing crime and violence and improving the quality of life in different areas of the world. One demonstration project was conducted in 1993 in Washington, DC, by Dr. John Hagelin and colleagues. An independent panel of more than twenty sociologists, criminologists, and members of the Washington, DC, government and police department advised on the study design and reviewed the analysis of the findings. The study included over 4000 people gathered in Washington to participate in a "peace assembly," practicing TM and specific related advanced programs for extended periods. Results showed that as the group size increased, there was a *highly significant decrease* in violent crime (32).

A remarkable aspect of this study was that it took place in August, when the weather is very hot in Washington, DC.

In fact, the police chief of Washington, who sat on the independent board of researchers monitoring the project, was quoted on the radio as saying, "The only way this group can lower crime by 20 percent in Washington in August is if we have two feet of snow!" In fact, the meditating group lowered crime by 23.6 percent.

How did this happen? The individuals in the group didn't go out on the streets and stop people from committing crimes. They simply meditated quietly together in various locations around the city. *The coherence effect they created in the collective consciousness of the city was like the result of throwing a pebble in a pond: ripples went out in all directions, creating sufficient coherence in the collective consciousness of the city so that crime was spontaneously reduced.*

What is the collective consciousness of a society?

The *collective consciousness* of a society is composed of the thoughts and feelings of all the individuals in that society. The concept of a collective consciousness underlying and influencing the structure of society has been expressed by many great thinkers in the past. William James, in his book *The Varieties of Religious Experience*, beautifully describes a shared level of collective consciousness in the following passage:

> Out of my experience, such as it is (and it is limited enough), one fixed conclusion dogmatically emerges, and that is this, that we with our lives are like islands in the

sea or like trees in the forest. The maple and the pine may whisper to each other with their leaves and Connecticut and Newport hear each other's foghorns. But the trees also commingle their roots in the darkness underground and the islands also hang together through the ocean's bottom.

Just so there is a continuum of cosmic consciousness against which our several minds plunge, as into a mother sea or reservoir.

Collective consciousness has never been studied in a serious scientific manner precisely *because* it could neither be isolated nor experimentally experienced. The most sophisticated sociological theories give a vague description, at best, of a social field as an interlocking network of social and behavioral interactions within specific economic and environmental conditions.

Research clearly demonstrates that it is possible to influence the collective consciousness of society through the group practice of the TM technique and its advanced programs.

Why hasn't government accepted this research and implemented these programs?

An interesting study that helped explain why this research has been ignored by government was conducted by Dr. Carla Brown as part of her doctoral thesis at Harvard University. Her research examined how five different groups of elite members of the Middle East policy community—peer reviewers, newspaper reporters, nongovernmental experts, and US diplomats and government officials—assessed one of the key published studies on the Maharishi Effect (33). This study showed that violence between nations could be reduced by the group practice of TM and its advanced programs. Most of the different groups in Washington who reviewed the results of this study, however, rejected it without even examining its scientific merit.

Dr. Brown's research suggested the existence of prejudice against research findings that did not conform to the belief system of the reviewers. This paradigm bias may be one of the important reasons governments have not yet been able to seriously consider and make use of these important findings.

Is there any hope that this research will someday be recognized and used by governments?

According to Maharishi, the leaders of any country reflect the collective consciousness of their country's people. In order for the leaders to make correct decisions, there must be coherence within the collective consciousness. Maharishi's solution was to inspire individuals in every country to organize large groups to regularly practice the TM technique and its advanced programs together. In this way, the collective consciousness will become coherent, and government will eventually acknowledge these research findings and support the implementation of these programs.

Chapter 7

The Brain, Consciousness, and Enlightenment

For thousands of years, men and women have tried to understand the nature of consciousness and the meaning of life. The axiom of the Greek philosopher Socrates, considered to be the grandfather of Western thought, was "Know thyself."

In this chapter, we'll explore how modern science deals with the age-old quest to know ourselves, and why TM is vital for a complete understanding of the nature of consciousness.

We'll also look at the state of consciousness called *enlightenment*. For centuries, the quest for enlightenment has captured the hearts and minds of seekers of knowledge. But the means to achieve it has been lost and revived countless times throughout the ages. Is it possible for anyone from any country or walk of life to achieve enlightenment? And can TM help in this quest?

What does science say about the nature of consciousness?

Science attempts to understand consciousness by understanding the parts of the brain. It asks questions like "What are the anatomical structures involved in emotions?" and "How can we define mental health in terms of the balance of specific chemicals in the brain?" Most neurophysiologists feel that given sufficient time and money, these questions can be answered in modern scientific, mechanistic terms. The answers, however, do not tell us about consciousness.

Philosophers and scientists have referred to the understanding of the true nature of consciousness as the "hard problem." And in all of history up to now, no one has been able to give a satisfactory answer as to what consciousness really is. The TM technique offers a solution to this dilemma by giving scientists a reliable tool with which to repeatedly explore consciousness in its most fundamental state, both experientially and in the lab.

How can we understand
the nature of consciousness?

Maharishi Mahesh Yogi developed a science and technology of consciousness, and the experimental basis of this new science is the practice of Transcendental Meditation. By directly experiencing consciousness through TM, refine and optimize the functioning of the human nervous system. We can use it as a kind of instrument to look within and to directly experience consciousness as the source of all thought and creativity.

What you, your neighbor, and all of us consider to be "normal" waking consciousness is in fact an extremely limited experience of the full potential of consciousness. The practice of TM enables us to experience consciousness in its simplest and purest state. And the development of higher states of consciousness provides us with a complete understanding of the true nature of consciousness, resulting in a state that is traditionally understood as enlightenment.

What is enlightenment?

Enlightenment has been misunderstood for many hundreds of years, in both the East and West, and has even been considered to be a state of self-delusion or self-denial. Maharishi has revised, clarified, and vastly enriched our knowledge about this state. We now know that the state of enlightenment represents the ultimate development of life: the ability to use 100 percent of our human potential. It is real and natural, and it develops systematically in a continuous and progressive manner on the basis of neurophysiological refinement until we at last reach higher states of consciousness.

This process of refinement uses the existing mechanics of our physiology to free both our mind and body from stress. Through the practice of TM, the process of the development of higher states of consciousness and full enlightenment is available to anyone, starting from any level of consciousness and without requiring any special lifestyle or system of belief. The ability to gain enlightenment is innate in every human being, and therefore, every human being deserves to have this experience. "There is no reason today in our scientific age," Maharishi said, "for anyone to remain unenlightened."

Are there any records of enlightenment?

The knowledge of enlightenment is an essential part of many ancient traditions. Maharishi explained that enlightenment and higher states of consciousness were well known in the ancient Vedic tradition but that "due to the long lapse of time," this knowledge was gradually lost, except to a handful of individuals.

Once the original, simple, systematic, and effective methods were lost, there arose in their place an enormous variety of less effective and more difficult techniques. Meditation procedures lost their once universal character and were replaced by austere practices of renunciation and detachment. Over millennia, the high regard that had once been accorded to higher states of consciousness and to the state of enlightenment was replaced by error, suspicion, and disbelief.

Are there any accounts of individuals achieving enlightenment in the West?

Enlightenment is a basic human experience, not owned by any single country or tradition. And although the systematic procedure for transcending intellectual thought and achieving the state of enlightenment was lost, nevertheless, there are many wonderful examples and written descriptions of men and women who have spontaneously glimpsed the state of enlightenment.

For example, in his masterwork, *Meditations*, Marcus Aurelius writes:

> Man seeks seclusion in the wilderness, by the seashore, or in the mountains—a dream you have cherished only too fondly yourself. But such fancies are wholly unworthy of a philosopher since at any moment you choose, you can retire within yourself. Nowhere can man find a quieter or more untroubled retreat than in his own soul; above all, he who possesses resources in himself, which he need only contemplate to secure immediate ease of mind. . . . Avail yourself often, then, of this retirement, and continually renew yourself.

An elegant account is given by Alfred, Lord Tennyson:

> All at once, as it were out of the intensity of the consciousness of individuality, individuality itself seemed to dissolve and fade away into boundless being, and this not a confused state but the clearest of the clear, the surest of the sure, utterly beyond words—where death was an almost laughable impossibility—the loss of personality (if so it were) seemed no extinction, but the only true self. I am

ashamed of my feeble description. Have I not said the state is utterly beyond words?

In his poem "Tintern Abbey," William Wordsworth gives a vivid description of the experience of transcending, even using physiological terms to characterize the state:

> —that serene and blessed mood,
> In which the affections gently lead us on—
> Until, the breath of this corporeal frame
> And even the motion of our human blood
> Almost suspended, we are laid asleep
> In body, and become a living soul:
> While with an eye made quiet by the power
> Of harmony, and the deep power of joy,
> We see into the life of things.

Besides philosophers and poets, have any modern scientists described experiences of transcending?

Perhaps one of the richest descriptions of transcendence has been given by Albert Einstein:

> There are moments when one feels free from one's own identification with human limitations and inadequacies. At such moments, one imagines that one stands on some spot of a small planet gazing in amazement at the cold yet profoundly moving beauty of the eternal, the unfathomable. Life and death flow into one, and there is neither evolution nor destiny, only Being.

These experiences are only a few of those recorded in our Western tradition. Enlightenment has been misunderstood for many hundreds of years, in both the East and West, and has even been considered to be a state of self-delusion or self-denial. Maharishi has revised, clarified, and vastly enriched our knowledge about this state. We now know that the state of enlightenment represents the ultimate development of life: the ability to use 100 percent of our human potential. It is real and natural, and it develops systematically in a continuous and progressive manner on the basis of neurophysiological refinement until we at last reach higher states of consciousness.

This process of refinement uses the existing mechanics of our physiology to free both our mind and body from stress. Through the practice of TM, the process of the development of higher states of consciousness and full enlightenment is available to anyone, starting from any level of consciousness and without requiring any special lifestyle or system of belief. The ability to gain enlightenment is innate in every human being, and therefore, every human being deserves to have this experience. "There is no reason today in our scientific age," Maharishi said, "for anyone to remain unenlightened."

How did this knowledge become lost?

Maharishi explains that this knowledge—and the practices with which to gain it—were lost not once but many times.

It is precisely because the experience of enlightenment depends upon a unique physiological state that it becomes difficult to achieve when the technology for gaining it easily becomes lost or forgotten. Because the human nervous system is an exceedingly delicate instrument, with many possible physiological states, neither verbal nor written instructions were sufficient to preserve the more subtle aspects of the knowledge.

The ability to experience pure consciousness is an innate capacity, like the ability to speak a language. However, in order to learn a language, a person must have the experience of speaking it. In order to directly experience pure consciousness, a person must learn how to transcend and reach subtler and subtler levels of thinking. What has been missing is this opportunity to learn how to systematically transcend and thereby cultivate higher states of consciousness.

Why is this knowledge available to us now?

In our age, we have been extremely fortunate to have Maharishi and his teacher, Guru Dev, both of whom lived the highest states of consciousness for the greater part of their lives and understood exactly what was needed to achieve these states. For an individual to spontaneously have experiences of transcending is not enough. A systematic and effective procedure is necessary in order to have *repeated experiences of transcending and develop higher states of consciousness.*

This is the knowledge that has been revived by Maharishi in its completeness and made available to us in the language of our time: the language of science. What Maharishi accomplished may be nothing less than the most important scientific discovery of our age. It heralds the exploration of the greatest frontier of modern science—the understanding and practical application of the science of consciousness. The practical application of this knowledge offers a unique opportunity to unfold the full potential of each individual and to create lasting peace and harmony in our precious world.

About the Authors

ROBERT KEITH WALLACE is a pioneering researcher on the physiology of consciousness. His work has inspired hundreds of studies on the benefits of meditation and other mind-body techniques. Dr. Wallace's findings have been published in *Science, American Journal of Physiology,* and *Scientific American.* He received his BS in physics and his PhD in physiology from UCLA, and he conducted postgraduate research at Harvard University. As the founding president of Maharishi University of Management (MUM) in Fairfield, Iowa, Dr. Wallace is currently Co-Dean of the College of Perfect Health, Professor and Chairman of the Department of Physiology and Health, and a Trustee of MUM.

Other books by Dr. Wallace include *Transcendental Meditation, Maharishi Ayurveda and Vedic Technology, The Neurophysiology of Enlightenment, Dharma Health and Beauty* (with Samantha Wallace), and *Dharma Parenting* (with Fred Travis).

LINCOLN AKIN NORTON is an entrepreneur, writer, and teacher of Transcendental Meditation. He started TM in 1966 while at Harvard and became a teacher in 1969. Since then he has served in numerous roles within the TM organization, including hosting one of the first TM for Business conferences with Maharishi Mahesh Yogi in 1976 at the Absolute Theory of Management Conference in Lausanne, Switzerland.

In 1982, he founded and became the CEO and Chairman of HRSoft, Inc., the first company to automate the mission-critical business area of Succession Planning and Management Development for the PC. Lincoln Norton was also the Founder and Chairman of the Corporate University, Inc., a membership organization that evaluated the best of the best of development activities for managers and executives in large companies around the world. In addition, he was a Founding Partner and Chairman of the Architectural Review Committee at Hartley Farms in Harding Township, New Jersey, an environmentally sensitive residential development that has won national acclaim for its innovative use of open spaces, architectural guidelines, and historic preservation.

References

1. Wallace, R.K. et al. A wakeful hypometabolic physiologic state. *American Journal of Physiology* 221(3): 795-799, 1971

• Dillbeck M.C. and Orme-Johnson D.W. Physiological differences between Transcendental Meditation and rest. *American Psychologist* 42:879–881, 1987

2. Travis, F.T. and Shear, J. Focused attention, open monitoring and automatic self-transcending: Categories to organize meditations from Vedic, Buddhist and Chinese traditions. *Consciousness and Cognition* 19(4):1110-1118, 2010

3. Travis F.T. and Arenander A. Cross-sectional and longitudinal study of effects of Transcendental Meditation practice on interhemispheric frontal asymmetry and frontal coherence. *International Journal of Neuroscience* 116:1519-1538, 2006

4. Orme-Johnson D.W. and Haynes C.T. EEG phase coherence, pure consciousness, creativity, and TM-Sidhi experiences. *International Journal of Neuroscience* 13: 211–217, 1981

5. Schneider R.H., et al. Stress Reduction in the Secondary Prevention of Cardiovascular Disease: Randomized, Controlled Trial of Transcendental Meditation and Health Education in Blacks. *Circ Cardiovasc Qual Outcomes* 5:750-758, 2012

• Jayadevappa R., et al. Effectiveness of Transcendental Meditation on functional capacity and quality of life of African Americans with congestive heart failure: a randomized control study. *Ethnicity and Disease* 17: 72-77, 2007

• Castillo-Richmond A., et al. Effects of the Transcendental Meditation Program on carotid atherosclerosis in hypertensive African Americans, *Stroke* 31: 568-573, 2000

• Kondwani K., Schneider R.H., Alexander C., Sledge C., Staggers F., Clayborne B., Sheppard W., Rainforth M., Krouse L., Orme-Johnson D. Left Ventricular Mass Regression with the Transcendental Meditation Technique and a Health Education Program in Hypertensive African Americans. *Journal of Social Behavior and Personality* 17:181-200, 2005

• Schneider R.H., Alexander C., Salerno J., Rainforth M., Nidich S. Stress Reduction in the Prevention and Treatment of Cardiovascular Disease in High Risk Underserved Populations: A Review of Controlled Research on the Transcendental Meditation Program. *Journal of Social Behavior and Personality* 17:159-180, 2005

• Zammara J. W., et al. Usefulness of the Transcendental Meditation program in the treatment of patients with coronary artery disease. *American Journal of Cardiology* 77: 867-870, 1996

6. Brook R.D. et al., Beyond Medications and Diet: Alternative Approaches to Lowering Blood Pressure. A Scientific Statement from the American Heart Association. *Hypertension* 61(6):1360-83, 2013

• Anderson J.W., et al. Blood pressure response to Transcendental Meditation: a meta-analysis. *American Journal of Hypertension* 21 (3): 310-316, 2008

• Barnes V.A., et al. Impact of Transcendental Meditation on ambulatory blood pressure in African-American adolescents. *American Journal of Hypertension* 17: 366-369, 2004

• Barnes V. A., et al. Stress, stress reduction, and hypertension in African Americans. *Journal of the National Medical Association* 89, 464-476, 1997

• Barnes V. A., et al. Acute effects of Transcendental Meditation on hemodynamic functioning in middle-aged adults. *Psychosomatic Medicine* 61 (4): 525-531, 1999

• Rainforth M.V., et al. Stress reduction programs in patients with elevated blood pressure: a systematic review and meta-analysis. *Current Hypertension Reports* 9:520–528, 2007

• Schneider R.H., et al. A randomized controlled trial of stress reduction in the treatment of hypertension in African Americans during one year. *American Journal of Hypertension* 18(1): 88-98, 2005

• Barnes V.A., and Orme-Johnson D. W. Clinical and Pre-clinical Applications of the Transcendental Meditation Program® in the Prevention and Treatment of Essential Hypertension and Cardiovascular Disease in Youth and Adults: A Research Review. *Current Hypertension Reviews* 2:207-218, 2006

• Herron, R.E., et al. Cost-Effective Hypertension Management: Comparison of Drug Therapies with an Alternative Program. *American Journal of Managed Care* Vol. II(4): 427–437, 1996

7. Cooper M. J., et al. Transcendental Meditation in the management of hypercholesterolemia. *Journal of Human Stress* 5(4): 24–27, 1979

• Cooper M. J. and Aygen M. M. Effect of Transcendental Meditation on serum cholesterol and blood pressure. Harefuah, *Journal of the Israel Medical Association* 95(1): 1-2, 1978

• Royer A. The role of the Transcendental Meditation technique in promoting smoking cessation: A longitudinal study. *Alcoholism Treatment Quarterly* 11: 219-236, 1994

8. Orme-Johnson D.W. Autonomic stability and Transcendental Meditation. *Psychosomatic Medicine* 35: 341-349, 1973

• Orme-Johnson D.W. and Walton K. W. All approaches of preventing or reversing effects of stress are not the same. *American Journal of Health Promotion* 12:297-299, 1998

• Barnes V. A., et al. Impact of Transcendental Meditation on cardiovascular function at rest and during acute stress in adolescents with high normal blood pressure. *Journal of Psychosomatic Research* 51: 597-605, 2001

• Gaylord C., et al. The effects of the Transcendental Meditation technique and progressive muscle relaxation on EEG coherence, stress reactivity, and mental health in black adults. *International Journal of Neuroscience* 46: 77-86, 1989

• Jevning R., et al. The transcendental meditation technique, adrenocortical activity, and implications for stress. *Experientia* 34(5): 618-619,1978

• Jevning R., et al. Adrenocortical activity during meditation, *Hormonal Behavior* 10(1):54-60, 1978

9. Paul-Labrador M., et al. Effects of randomized controlled trial of Transcendental Meditation on components of the metabolic syndrome

in subjects with coronary heart disease. *Archives of Internal Medicine* 166:1218-1224, 2006

10. DavidLynchFoundation.org

11. Wilson A.F. et al. Transcendental Meditation and asthma. *Respiration* 32:74-80, 1975

• Haratani T., et al. Effects of Transcendental Meditation (TM) on the mental health of industrial workers. *Japanese Journal of Industrial Health* 32: 656, 1990

• Orme-Johnson D. W., et al. Meditation in the treatment of chronic pain and insomnia. In National Institutes of Health Technology Assessment Conference on Integration of Behavioral and Relaxation Approaches into the Treatment of Chronic Pain and Insomnia, Bethesda Maryland: National Institutes of Health, 1995

• Orme-Johnson D.W, et al. Neuroimaging of meditation's effect on brain reactivity to pain. *NeuroReport* 17(12):1359-63, 2006

• Mills W. W. and Farrow J. T. The Transcendental Meditation technique and acute experimental pain. *Psychosomatic Medicine* 43(2): 157–164, 1981

• Alexander C.N., et al. Treating and preventing alcohol, nicotine, and drug abuse through Transcendental Meditation: A review and statistical meta-analysis. *Alcoholism Treatment Quarterly* 11: 13-87, 1994.

• Orme-Johnson D. W. Transcendental Meditation as an epidemiological approach to drug and alcohol abuse: Theory, research, and financial impact evaluation. *Alcoholism Treatment Quarterly* 11: 119-165, 1994

• Walton K.G., and Levitsky, D.A. A neuroendocrine mechanism for the reduction of drug use and addictions by Transcendental Meditation. *Alcoholism Treatment Quarterly* 11: 89-117, 1994

12. Nidich S., Fields J., Rainforth M., Pomerantz R., Cella D., Kristeller J., Salerno J., Schneider R.H. A Randomized Controlled Trial of the Effects of Transcendental Meditation on Quality of Life in Older Breast Cancer Patients. *Integrative Cancer Therapies* 8(3): 228-234, 2009

13. Orme-Johnson D.W. Medical Care Utilization and the Transcendental Meditation Program. *Psychosomatic Medicine* 49: 493–507, 1987

• Orme-Johnson D. W., Herron R. E. An Innovative Approach to Reducing Medical Care Utilization and Expenditures. *American Journal of Managed Care* 3: 135–144,1997

14. Herron R.E., et al. The Impact of the Transcendental Meditation Program on Government Payments to Physicians in Quebec. *American Journal of Health Promotion* 10: 208–216, 1996

• Herron, R.E., Hillis, S. L. The Impact of the Transcendental Meditation Program on Government Payments to Physicians in Quebec: An Update. *American Journal of Health Promotion* 14(5): 284–291, 2000

• Herron R.E. Can the Transcendental Meditation Program Reduce the Medical Expenditures of Older People? A Longitudinal Cost-Reduction Study in Canada. *Journal of Social Behavior and Personality* 17(1): 415–442, 2005

• Herron, R.E. Changes in Physician Costs Among High-Cost Transcendental Meditation Practitioners Compared with High-Cost Non-practitioners Over 5 Years. *American Journal of Health Promotion* 26(1): 56–60, 2011

15 Brooks J.S. and Scarano T. Transcendental Meditation in the treatment of post-Vietnam adjustment. *Journal of Counseling and Development* 64: 212-215, 1985

16. Duraimani S. et al. Effects of Lifestyle Modification on Telomerase Gene Expression in Hypertensive Patients: A Pilot Trial of Stress Reduction and Health Education Programs in African Americans. *PLOS ONE* 10(11): e0142689, 2015

• Wenuganen, S. Anti-Aging Effects of the Transcendental Meditation Program: Analysis of Ojas Level and Global Gene Expression Maharishi University of Management, ProQuest Dissertations Publishing, 3630467, 2014

17. Barnes V.A., et al. Impact of Transcendental Meditation on mortality in older African Americans—eight year follow-up. *Journal of Social Behavior and Personality* 17(1): 201-216, 2005

• Glaser J.L., et al. Elevated serum dehydroepiandrosterone sulfate levels in practitioners of the Transcendental Meditation (TM) and TM-Sidhi programs. *Journal of Behavioral Medicine* 15: 327-341, 1992

• Schneider R.H., et al. The Transcendental Meditation program: reducing the risk of heart disease and mortality and improving quality of life in African Americans. *Ethnicity and Disease* 11: 159-60, 2001

• Schneider R.H., et al. Long-term effects of stress reduction on mortality in persons > 55 years of age with systemic hypertension. *American Journal of Cardiology* 95: 1060-1064, 2005

18. Wallace R.K., et al. The effects of the Transcendental Meditation and TM-Sidhi program on the aging process. *International Journal of Neuroscience* 16: 53-58, 1982

19. Alexander C.N., et al. Transcendental Meditation, mindfulness, and longevity. *Journal of Personality and Social Psychology* 57: 950-964, 1989

• Alexander C.N., et al. The effects of Transcendental Meditation compared to other methods of relaxation in reducing risk factors, morbidity, and mortality. *Homeostasis* 35: 243-264, 1994

20. Eppley K.R. et al. Differential effects of relaxation techniques on trait anxiety: A meta-analysis. *Journal of Clinical Psychology* 45: 957-974, 1989

21. Orme-Johnson, D.W., & Barnes, V.A. Effects of the Transcendental Meditation technique on Trait Anxiety: A Meta-Analysis of Randomized Controlled Trials. *Journal of Alternative and Complementary Medicine* 19: 1-12, 2013

• Alexander C.N., et al. Effects of the Transcendental Meditation program on stress reduction, health, and employee development: A prospective study in two occupational settings. *Anxiety, Stress and Coping: An International Journal* 6: 245-262, 1993

• Kniffki C. Tranzendentale Meditation und Autogenes Training- Ein Vergleich (Transcendental Meditation and Autogenic Training: A Comparison). Munich: Kindler *Verlag Geist und Psyche,* 1979

• Geisler M. Therapeutiche Wirkungen der Transzendentalen Meditation auf drogenkonsumenten (Therapeutic effects of Transcendental Meditation on drug use). *Zeitschrift fur Klinische Psychologie* 7: 235-255, 1978

• Ferguson P.C., et al. Psychological Findings on Transcendental Meditation. *Journal of Humanistic Psychology* 16: 483-488, 1976

References

• Candelent T., et al. Teaching Transcendental Meditation in a psychiatric setting. *Hospital & Community Psychiatry* 26: 156-159, 1975

• Dillbeck M.C. The effect of the Transcendental Meditation technique on anxiety level. *Journal of Clinical Psychology* 33: 1076-1078, 1977

• Ljunggren G. Inflytandet av Transcendental Meditation pa neuroticism, medicinbruk och sömnproblem. *Läkartidningen* 74(47): 4212–4214, 1977

• Lovell-Smith H. D. Transcendental Meditation—treating the patient as well as the disease. *The New Zealand Family Physician* 9: 62–65, 1982

• Tjoa A. Increased intelligence and reduced neuroticism through the Transcendental Meditation program. *Gedrag: Tijdschrift voor Psychologie* 3: 167-182, 1975

• Alexander C.N., et al. Transcendental Meditation, self-actualization, and psychological health: A conceptual overview and statistical meta-analysis. *Journal of Social Behavior and Personality* 6: 189-247, 1991

• Gelderloos P. Cognitive orientation toward positive values in advanced participants of the TM and TM-Sidhi program. *Perceptual and Motor Skills* 64: 1003-1012, 1987

• Gelderloos P., et al. Transcendence and psychological health: studies with long-term participants of the Transcendental Meditation and TM-Sidhi program. *Journal of Psychology* 124(2): 177–197, 1990

• Jedraczak A. The Transcendental Meditation and TM-Sidhi program and field independence. *Perceptual and Motor Skills* 59: 999-100, 1984

• Nidich S., et al. Influence of Transcendental Meditation: A replication. *Journal of Counseling Psychology* 20: 565-566, 1973

• Pelletier K.R. Influence of Transcendental Meditation upon autokinetic perception. *Perceptual and Motor Skills* 39: 1031-1034, 1974

• Seeman W., et al. Influence of Transcendental Meditation on a measure of self-actualization. *Journal of Counseling Psychology* 19: 184-187, 1972

• Nidich S. et al. Moral Development and Higher States of Consciousness. *Journal of Adult Developement* 7(4): 217-255, 2000

22. Broome R., et al. Worksite stress reduction through the Transcendental Meditation Program. *Journal of Social Behavior and Personality* 17(1): 235–276, 2005

• Frew D.R. Transcendental Meditation and productivity. *Academy of Management Journal* 17: 362-368, 1974

• Harung H. S., et al. Peak performance and higher states of consciousness: A study of world-class performers. *Journal of Managerial Psychology* 11(4): 3–23, 1996

• Schmidt-Wilk J. Consciousness-based management development: Case studies of international top management teams. *Journal of Transnational Management Development* 5(3): 61–85, 2000

• Alexander C. N., et al. Effects of the Transcendental Meditation program on stress-reduction, health, and employee development: A prospective study in two occupational settings. *Stress, Anxiety and Coping* 6: 245–262, 1993

• Alexander C.N., et al. Promoting adult psychological development: Implications for management education. *Proceedings of the Association of Management, Human Resource Management* 2: 133–137, 1990

23. Wallace R.K. Physiological effects of Transcendental Meditation. *Science* 167:1751-1754, 1970

• Wallace, R.K. Physiological effects of the Transcendental Meditation technique: A proposed fourth major state of consciousness. Ph.D. thesis. Physiology Department, University of California, Los Angeles, 1970

• Alexander C.N. et al.. Transcendental consciousness: A fourth state of consciousness beyond sleep, dreaming and waking, in Gackenbach J. (Ed.): Sourcebook on Sleep and Dreams. New York, Garland, 1986

• Travis F.T., and Pearson C. Pure consciousness: distinct phenomenological and physiological correlates of 'Consciousness Itself'. *International Journal of Neuroscience* 100: 77-89, 2000

• Alexander C.N., et al. Transcendental consciousness: a fourth state of consciousness beyond sleep, dreaming, and waking. in J. Gackenbach (ed.), *Sleep and Dreams: A Sourcebook* New York: Garland Publishing, Inc., 282–315, 1986

• Travis F.T., Wallace R.K. Autonomic and EEG patterns during eyes-closed rest and Transcendental Meditation (TM) practice: a basis for a neural model of TM practice. *Consciousness and Cognition* 8: 302-318, 1999

References

• Travis F.T., Wallace R.K. Autonomic patterns during respiratory suspensions: possible markers of Transcendental Consciousness. *Psychophysiology* 34: 39-46, 1997

• Travis F.T. Autonomic and EEG patterns distinguish transcending from other experiences during Transcendental Meditation practice. *International Journal of Psychophysiology* 42: 1-9, 2001

24. Mason L.I. et al. Electrophysiological correlates of higher states of consciousness during sleep in long-term practitioners of the Transcendental Meditation program. *Sleep* 20: 102-110, 1997

• Travis F.T. From I to I: concepts of Self on an object-referral/ self-referral continuum. In AP Prescott (ed.), The Concept of Self in Psychology. New York: Nova Publishing, 2006

25.Travis F.T. et al. Patterns of EEG coherence, power and contingent negative variation characterize the integration of transcendental and waking states. *Biological Psychology* 61: 293-319, 2002

• Travis F., Haaga D., Hagelin J., Tanner M., Nidich S., Gaylord-King C., Grosswald S., Rainforth M., Schneider R.H. Effects of Transcendental Meditation Practice on Brain Functioning and Stress Reactivity in College Students. *International Journal of Psychophysiology* 71(2): 170-176, 2009

26. Cranson R.W., et al. Transcendental Meditation and improved performance on intelligence-related measures: A longitudinal study. *Personality and Individual Differences* 12: 1105-1116, 1991

• So K.T. and Orme-Johnson D.W. Three randomized experiments on the longitudinal effects of the Transcendental Meditation technique on cognition. *Intelligence* 29: 419-440, 2001

27. DavidLynchFoundation.org

28. Travis F.T. et al. ADHD, Brain Functioning, and Transcendental Meditation Practice Mind & Brain: *The Journal of Psychiatry* 2 (1): 73-81, 2011

29. Rosaen C, Benn R. The experience of transcendental meditation in middle school students: a qualitative report. *Explore* (NY). 2(5): 422-425, 2006

30. Travis F., Haaga D., Hagelin J., Tanner M., Nidich S., Gaylord-King C., Grosswald S., Rainforth M., Schneider R.H. Effects of Transcendental Meditation Practice on Brain Functioning and Stress Reactivity in College Students. *International Journal of Psychophysiology* 71(2):170-176, 2009

• Nidich S., Rainforth M., Haaga D., Hagelin J., Salerno J., Travis F., Tanner M., Gaylord- King C., Grosswald S., Schneider R. H. A Randomized Controlled Trial on Effects of the Transcendental Meditation Program on Blood Pressure, Psychological Distress, and Coping in Young Adults. *American Journal of Hypertension* 22(12): 1326-1331, 2009

• Haaga D., Grosswald S., Gaylord-King C., Rainforth M., Tanner M., Travis F., Nidich S., Schneider R.H. Effects of the Transcendental Meditation Program on Substance Use Among University Students. *Cardiology Research and Practice* 2011: 537101, 2011

31.Chandler H.M., et al. Transcendental Meditation and postconventional self-development: A 10-year longitudinal study. *Journal of Social Behavior and Personality* 17(1): 93–121, 2005

• Nidich S.I., et al. School effectiveness: Achievement gains at the Maharishi School of the Age of Enlightenment. *Education* 107: 49-54, 1986

• Nidich S.I. and Nidich R.J. Increased academic achievement at Maharishi School of the Age of Enlightenment: A replication study. *Education* 109: 302-304, 1989

• Gelderloos P. Field independence of students at Maharishi School of the Age of Enlightenment and a Montessori school. *Perceptual and Motor Skills* 65: 613-614, 1987

32. Hagelin J.S .et al. Effects of group practice of the Transcendental Meditation program on preventing violent crime in Washington, DC: results of the National Demonstration Project, June-July 1993. *Social Indicators Research* 47: 153-201, 1999

• Dillbeck, M.C. et al. The Transcendental Meditation program and crime rate change in a sample of forty-eight cities. *Journal of Crime and Justice* 4: 25–45, 1981

• Dillbeck, M.C. et al. Test of a field model of consciousness and social change: The Transcendental Meditation and TM-Sidhi program and decreased urban crime. *The Journal of Mind and Behavior* 9: 457–486, 1988

• Cavanaugh, K.L. Time series analysis of U.S. and Canadian inflation and unemployment: A test of a field-theoretic hypothesis. Proceedings of the American Statistical Association, Business and Economics Statistics Section (Alexandria, VA: American Statistical Association): 799–804, 1987

• Dillbeck, M.C. et al. Consciousness as a field: The Transcendental Meditation and TM-Sidhi program and changes in social indicators. *The Journal of Mind and Behavior* 8: 67–104, 1987

• Cavanaugh, K.L. and King, K.D. Simultaneous transfer function analysis of Okun's misery index: Improvements in the economic quality of life through Maharishi's Vedic Science and technology of consciousness. Proceedings of the American Statistical Association, Business and Economics Statistics Section (Alexandria, VA: American Statistical Association): 491–496, 1988

• Orme-Johnson, D.W. et al. International peace project in the Middle East: The effect of the Maharishi Technology of the Unified Field. *Journal of Conflict Resolution* 32: 776–812, 1988

• Davies, J.L. Alleviating political violence through enhancing coherence in collective consciousness. Dissertation Abstracts International 49(8): 2381A, 1989

• Dillbeck, M.C. Test of a field theory of consciousness and social change: Time series analysis of participation in the TM-Sidhi program and reduction of violent death in the U.S. *Social Indicators Research* 22: 399–418, 1990

• Gelderloos, P. et al. The dynamics of US–Soviet relations, 1979–1986: Effects of reducing social stress through the Transcendental Meditation and TM-Sidhi program. Proceedings of the Social Statistics Section of the American Statistical Association (Alexandria, VA: American Statistical Association): 297–302, 1990

• Assimakis, P.D. and Dillbeck, M.C. Time series analysis of improved quality of life in Canada: Social change, collective consciousness, and the TM-Sidhi program. *Psychological Reports* 76: 1171–1193, 1995

• Dillbeck, M.C. and Rainforth, M.V. Impact assessment analysis of behavioral quality of life indices: Effects of group practice of the Transcendental Meditation and TM-Sidhi program. Proceedings of the Social

Statistics Section of the American Statistical Association (Alexandria, VA: American Statistical Association): 38–43, 1996

• Hatchard, G.D. et al. A model for social improvement. Time series analysis of a phase transition to reduced crime in Merseyside metropolitan area. *Psychology, Crime, and Law* 2: 165–174, 1996

• Orme-Johnson, D.W., et al. Preventing terrorism and international conflict: Effects of large assemblies of participants in the Transcendental Meditation and TM-Sidhi programs. *Journal of Offender Rehabilitation* 36: 283–302, 2003

33. Brown C.L. Overcoming barriers to use of promising research among elite Middle East policy groups. *Journal of Social Behavior and Personality* 17:489-546, 2005

References

How to Learn TM: The Seven Steps

Introducing the Practice

Step 1: Introductory Lecture (45 minutes)
A vision of all possibilities through the Transcendental Meditation program

Step 2: Preparatory Lecture (20 minutes)
The mechanics and origin of the TM technique

Step 3: Personal Interview (10 to 15 minutes)
Interview with a certified teacher of the TM program, immediately following the Preparatory Lecture

Four Days of Instruction
(Held over four consecutive days)

Step 4: Personal Instruction (1 to 2 hours)
Learning the TM technique (one-on-one with a certified TM teacher)

Step 5: First Day of Checking (1 to 2 hours)

Verifying the correctness of the practice and further instruction

Step 6: Second Day of Checking (1 to 2 hours)

Understanding the mechanics of the TM technique based on personal experiences

Step 7: Third Day of Checking (1 to 2 hours)

Understanding the growth of higher states of consciousness

Your initial TM course fee gives you a lifelong learning program that includes personal follow-up meetings, monthly advanced knowledge meetings, and other events. To learn about your course fee for your age and country please go to TM.org.

TM Websites

Find a TM Teacher Anywhere in World

Starting TM—TM.org

Refer a friend —tmrefer.org

Information on TM

TM News—TM.org/blog

Enlightenment Magazine—TMMagazine.org

TM Media Alert—TM.org/Media-Alerts

Consciousness Talks—ConsciousnessTalks.org

Scientific Research

Research explained—TruthAboutTM.org

Advanced Programs

Advanced programs for meditators—Advanced.TM.org

Health

Ask the Doctors—AskTheDoctors.com

American Association of Health Professionals Practicing
TM—TMHealthConference.org

TM and autism—TM-Autism.org

Business

Center for Leadership Performance—TMBusiness.org

Peace

Global Union of Scientists for Peace—GUSP.org
International Center for Invincible Defense
—InvincibleDefense.org

Education

Maharishi University of Management—MUM.edu
Maharishi School—MSAE.edu

Programs for At-Risk Populations

At-Risk Populations—DavidLynchFoundation.org
Veterans—TM.org/tm-for-vets

Social Media

Facebook TM—Facebook.com/TM
meditation
LinkedIn TM Professionals—LinkedIn.com/
groups/1829032
Twitter TM—Twitter.com/TMmeditation
YouTube TM—YouTube.com/user/MeditationChannel

Contact the Publisher

Bulk orders — dharmapublications.com

Readings on TM

Transcendence: Healing and Transformation through Transcendental Meditation by Norman Rosenthal, Tarcher/ Perigee, 2012

Super Mind: How to Boost Performance and Live a Richer and Happier Life Through Transcendental Meditation by Norman Rosenthal, Tarcher/Perigee, 2016

Transcendental Meditation: Revised and Updated by Robert Roth, Primus, 1994

Science of Being and Art of Living: Transcendental Meditation by Maharishi Mahesh Yogi, Plume, 2001

Catching the Big Fish: Meditation, Consciousness, and Creativity by David Lynch, Tarcher/Penguin, 2007

Transcendental Meditation: A Scientist's Journey to Happiness, Health, and Peace, Adapted and Updated from The Physiology of Consciousness: Part I by Robert Keith Wallace, PhD, Dharma Publications, 2016

The Neurophysiology of Enlightenment: How Maharishi's Transcendental Meditation and TM-Sidhi Program Transform the Functioning of the Human Body, Updated and Revised by Robert Keith Wallace, PhD, Dharma Publications, 2016

Dharma Parenting: Understand Your Child's Brilliant Brain for Greater Happiness, Health, Success, and Fulfillment by Robert Keith Wallace PhD, and Fredrick Travis PhD, Tarcher/Perigee, 2016

Maharishi Ayurveda and Vedic Technology: Creating Ideal Health for the Individual and World, Revised and Updated from The Physiology of Consciousness: Part 2 by Robert Keith Wallace, PhD, Dharma Publications, 2016

Dharma Health and Beauty: A User-Friendly Introduction to Ayurveda, Book One of the Smith Family Saga by Samantha Wallace with Robert Keith Wallace, PhD, Dharma Publications, 2016

A Simple Glossary of Terms

Consciousness: Consciousness is the quality of being awake or aware. Our state of consciousness fluctuates, depending on the state of our physiology (how well we have slept in the night, what we've eaten, etc.).

Pure Consciousness: The experience of consciousness in its simplest, most fundamental state, devoid of thought content (and hence without boundaries) and wide awake to its own nature.

Finer levels of thinking: If we consider the mind to be like an ocean, with a very active surface level and a more silent, deep level, then "finer levels of thinking" are what we experience when the mind settles down from its active surface to quieter and deeper levels.

Mantra: An ancient sound or vibration, which has only good effects on both the mind and body. Its importance lies in its sound value, rather than meaning, and it's used to allow the mind to follow its natural tendency to "transcend" to fields of greater happiness.

Transcending: The effortless settling down of the mind during TM practice from its surface activity to finer and finer levels of thinking and ultimately to the source of thought, pure consciousness.

Transcendence: The experience of pure consciousness, when our awareness goes beyond, or transcends, all mental activity.

Normal states of consciousness: These are the three basic states of consciousness, known to everybody as waking, dreaming, and sleeping. Each has its own unique physiological correlates.

Transcendental Consciousness: The fourth state of consciousness, which is completely different from waking, dreaming, and sleeping. We experience this state by transcending mental activity and gaining access to the source of thought, pure consciousness, the unified field of consciousness. The physiological markers of Transcendental Consciousness include EEG coherence and quiescent breathing—indicators of a unique state of "restful alertness."

Cosmic Consciousness: This state of consciousness is the fifth state, and is cultivated through regular practice of Transcendental Meditation alternated with daily activity. It is characterized by the permanent co-existence of pure consciousness with waking, dreaming, and sleeping states. It becomes stabilized when all stresses in the nervous system have dissolved and the system is functioning normally.

Refined Cosmic Consciousness: This state of consciousness is the sixth state, which comes about naturally when someone has lived in the fifth state for some time. Sometimes called God Consciousness, it becomes established through the progressive refinement of perception until one can perceive the full range of creation, from its surface values to its deepest level—an experience that gives rise to profound appreciation and love for the perfection and beauty of nature.

Unity Consciousness: This is the seventh and highest state of consciousness in Maharishi's description of states of consciousness. In this state everything, close and far, is experienced in terms of the unbounded innermost Self.

The Maharishi Effect: Scientists have shown that one percent of a population practicing the Transcendental Meditation technique there are measurable improvements in the quality of life for the whole population.

The Extended Maharishi Effect: Scientists found that when even the square root of one percent of any population practices the TM and more advanced TM-Sidhi programs in a group, there is a measurable, marked reduction in violence and an improvement in the quality of life.

Acknowledgments

We would like to acknowledge Gerry Geer his excellent final editing, Jennifer Hawthorne for her work on an earlier version of the book, and Samantha Wallace for all her brilliant help and inspiration. We thank Allen Cobb for helping to prepare this book and George Foster for his wonderful cover designs. Thanks to Sam Katz and Dennis Rowe for their lively suggestions.

Index

A

B

C

D

E

education 15, 55, 59
EEG 90, 91
EEG coherence 91
emotions 72
enlightenment 15, 71, 73, 74, 75

G

gamma 22
Guru Dev 78

H

Hagelin, John 66
happiness 13, 14, 40, 103
hard problem 72
health 15, 16, 37, 40, 41, 44, 45, 47, 72
health care costs 41
heart disease 38, 39, 40
high blood pressure 37, 39, 40
higher states of consciousness 15, 47, 49, 52, 74, 78, 98

I

insomnia 40, 42
insulin resistance 40
intelligence 14, 55
IQ 56

J

James, William 67

L

longevity 44, 45
long-term practice of TM 47
Lynch, David 58, 59, 101

M

Maharishi 29, 52, 61, 65, 66, 69, 72, 74, 78, 79, 81, 82, 87, 101, 102
Maharishi Effect 66
Maharishi University of Management 81, 87